Haifa Bradai
Sondes Laajimi
Rabeb Mbarek

Heat stroke; North African experience

Haifa Bradai
Sondes Laajimi
Rabeb Mbarek

Heat stroke; North African experience

epidemioclinical and prognostic study of patients treated for heatstroke in the prehospital setting

ScienciaScripts

Imprint

Any brand names and product names mentioned in this book are subject to trademark, brand or patent protection and are trademarks or registered trademarks of their respective holders. The use of brand names, product names, common names, trade names, product descriptions etc. even without a particular marking in this work is in no way to be construed to mean that such names may be regarded as unrestricted in respect of trademark and brand protection legislation and could thus be used by anyone.

Cover image: www.ingimage.com

This book is a translation from the original published under ISBN 978-620-6-71929-8.

Publisher:
Sciencia Scripts
is a trademark of
Dodo Books Indian Ocean Ltd. and OmniScriptum S.R.L publishing group

120 High Road, East Finchley, London, N2 9ED, United Kingdom
Str. Armeneasca 28/1, office 1, Chisinau MD-2012, Republic of Moldova, Europe
Printed at: see last page
ISBN: 978-620-7-98794-8

CONTENTS

INTRODUCTION 4

MATERIALS AND METHOD 5

RESULTS 9

DISCUSSION..19

STRENGTHS AND LIMITATIONS OF THE STUDY 26

CONCLUSION 27

REFERENCES..29

APPENDICES...31

INTRODUCTION

Theat stroke is a life-threatening medical emergency (1). Clinically, it is defined by the combination of a rapid rise in core temperature above 40°C and neurological (delirium, convulsions or coma) and cardiovascular disorders. (2,3). An alternative definition of heatstroke is based on its pathophysiology and states that heatstroke is a form of hyperthermia associated with a systemic inflammatory response that leads to a syndrome of multivisceral dysfunction, principally encephalopathy (2).

In fact, there are two types of heatstroke, depending on the presence or absence of exertion. The first type is exertional heatstroke, which develops in active individuals such as athletes, soldiers or workers performing rigorous physical activities (3,4).

The second type is classic heatstroke without effort. This type of heatstroke occurs at rest following excessive exposure to heat, leading to thermoregulatory failure. It develops in most cases in ambulant elderly people with co-morbidities including obesity, diabetes, hypertension, heart disease, renal failure, dementia and alcoholism (3,4). Our study describes the characteristics of this type of heatstroke. Despite improvements in cooling techniques and the therapeutic management of heatstroke victims, the risk of progression to multi-visceral failure and the mortality rate remain high (2).

The aim of our work is to :
- To describe the clinical, therapeutic and prognostic features of heatstroke in 27 cases treated in a pre-hospital setting.

- Determine predictive factors for mortality using univariate analysis.

MATERIALS AND METHOD

I. Type of study

Our work is a descriptive cross-sectional study conducted by the SAMU 03 service in the centre-east (four governorates: Mahdia, Monastir, Sousse and Kairouan) over a period of 3 months (June-August 2023).

II. Study population

Our study population consisted of 27 heatstroke victims treated by SAMU03 teams during the summer heatwave of 2023.

Inclusion criteria :

- Age $\geq$ 18 years
- Any call for non-strenuous heatstroke occurring at rest.

Exclusion criteria :

- Age < 18
- Any call for exercise heat stroke.

III. Data collection

The information was collected using a specific form which takes into account the epidemiological, clinical, therapeutic and prognostic data of the patients (Appendix 1).

1. Epidemiological data

Date and time of call, ambient temperature at time of call. Data related to the mission: Governorate of the call (Sousse, Monastir, Kairouan, Mahdia),

Regulation decision: to engage the team or not, SMUR engaged (Kairouan, Sousse, Monastir, Mahdia, Jam), Reason for the call (disorders of consciousness, dyspnoea, haemodynamic instability), type of mission (primary, primary-secondary, secondary), place of intervention (home, public place, peripheral emergency).

Patient data: gender, age, medical history, daily physical activity, lifestyle habits: smoking, alcohol, obesity, average water consumption per 24 hours.

2. Clinical and biological data

- Symptomatology: general signs: fever, nausea/vomiting, fatigue, dizziness, cramps; signs of dehydration: sensation of thirst, dry skin; neurological signs: headache, confusion, coma, syncope.

- Clinical parameters on initial examination :

•Haemodynamics: blood pressure, heart rate, peripheral signs of shock, ECG.

•Respiratory plan: respiratory rate, saturation, work of breathing, auscultation.

•Neurological: Glasgow score (5) (appendix 2), state of pupils, signs of localisation, temperature, dextro

- Biology: CBC, haemostasis work-up: PT/INR, ionogram (natraemia, kalaemia), renal function, liver work-up (ASAT, ALAT, BT, BD), CPK, LDH.

3. Therapeutic management

- Duration of treatment:.... (in hours)

- CAT: Moving to a cooler place, Physical cooling, Pharmacological cooling, Oral hydration, Filling with cooled serum, Placing in PLS, Use of anti-inflammatories, Oxygen therapy, Respiratory assistance, Vasoactive drugs.

4. Evolution

- Regulation decision (referral): LSP or transfer to hospital.

- Improvement without sequelae, time to improvement (in hours):...

- Initial visceral damage (cerebral, cardiac, hepatic, renal, haematological)

- Sequels remaining (Cerebral, Cardiac Hepatic, Renal, Haematological)

- Duration of treatment before improvement: ... hours

- Duration of care before death: .... hours

IV. Statistical analysis of data

Statistical analysis was carried out using SPSS 21.0 statistical analysis software.

1. Descriptive section

Continuous variables were expressed as mean (± standard deviation) with minimum and maximum.

Qualitative variables were expressed as headcounts and percentages.

2. Analytical part

In this section, using a univariate analysis in the first instance, we compared patients who died as a result of heatstroke with those who did not, in relation to the different variables measured. The tests used were the Chi-2 test for comparing percentages and the Student's t test for comparing means. The significance level was set at 5%.

V.Definition of heat stroke

Heat stroke: There is no universally accepted definition of heat stroke. heat stroke. The most commonly used definition of heatstroke in the world is that of Bouchama (2).Bouchama defined heat stroke as the combination of a rapid rise in core temperature above 40°C and neurological disorders (delirium, convulsions or coma) (2). In Japan, the Japan Association for Acute Medicine (JAAM) has collected data via a national heat illness registry of patients diagnosed with heat illness (including heat stroke) regardless of core body temperature since 2006 (3,6) . The JAAM established and published criteria for heat-related illness, including heat stroke, in 2014 (3) (appendix 3).

Heat stroke has been defined as a patient exposed to high ambient temperature who meets one or more of the following criteria:

1. Central nervous system manifestations (altered consciousness with a score on the Japanese coma scale $\geq$ 2 (7) (appendix 4), cerebellar symptoms, convulsions or seizures)

2. Liver/kidney dysfunction (follow-up after hospitalisation, liver or kidney failure requiring hospital care);

3. Coagulation disorders [diagnosed as disseminated intravascular coagulation (DIC) by JAAM] (3,8,9) (appendix 5).

Body temperature has not been included in these diagnostic criteria due to several fatal cases of patients with body temperatures below 40°C observed in clinical practice (10) . In 2016, a working group of the JAAM Heat Stroke Committee (JAAM-HS-WG) simplified the classification of heat stroke (10). The modified JAAM definition of heat stroke included patients exposed to high environmental temperatures and meeting at least one of the following criteria:

1. Glasgow Coma Scale (GCS) score $\leq$ 14,

2. Creatinine or total bilirubin levels $\geq$ 1.2 mg/dL,

3. JAAM DIC (Disseminated Intravascular Coagulation) score $\geq$ 4.

The difference in the definitions/classifications of heat stroke between Bouchama's definition and the JAAM and JAAM-HS-WG criteria was illustrated in the table below (3)(appendix 6)

RESULTS

I. Descriptive study

1. Epidemiological data

1.1.Data related to heat stroke missions

1.1.1. Ambient temperature at the time of calls

The average ambient temperature during the calls was 32.5 ± 4.5°C, with an average maximum temperature of 39.8 ± 4.5°C and an average minimum temperature of 25.3 ± 3.5°C.

1.1.2. Breakdown of assignments by call governorate

Most calls to the Samu 03 came from the governorate of Sousse in 15 cases (55.5%), followed by the governorate of Monastir in 7 cases (25.9%), the governorate of Kairouan in 3 cases (11.1%) and the governorate of Mahdia in 2 cases (7.4%).

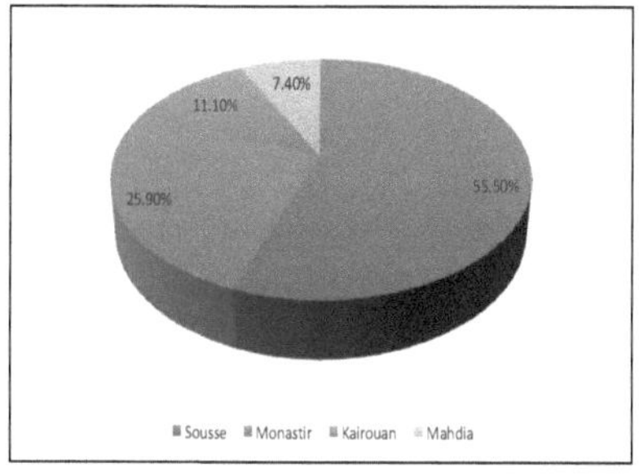

Figure 1: Breakdown of missions by call governorate

1.1.3. Breakdown of heat stroke missions

Depending on the reason for the call The reason for the call was disorders of consciousness in all cases, dyspnoea associated with disorders of consciousness in 4 cases (14.8%) and haemodynamic instability with disorders of consciousness in 6 cases (22.2%).

1.1.4. Breakdown of missions according to regulatory decision

Regulation decided to involve the team in 25 cases, i.e. 92.6%, and not to intervene in 2 cases, given the unavailability of resources in 1 case and an incomplete request in the second.

1.1.5. Breakdown of missions by type of SMUR involved

The table below shows the breakdown of missions by type of SMUR involved

Table I: Breakdown by type of SMUR involved:

	Workforce	Percentage (%)
SMUR Hached Sousse	8	29,6
SMUR Sahloul Sousse	7	25,9
SMUR Monastir	7	25,9
SMUR Kairouan	3	11,2
SMUR Mehdia	1	3,7
SMUR Jem	1	3,7
Total	27	100

1.1.6. Breakdown by type of assignment and location intervention

The type of mission was primary in 17 cases (63%) and primary-secondary in 8 cases (29.6%). The place of intervention was at home in 16 cases (59.3%), in a public place in 1 case (3.7%) and in an outlying emergency department in 8 cases (29.6%).

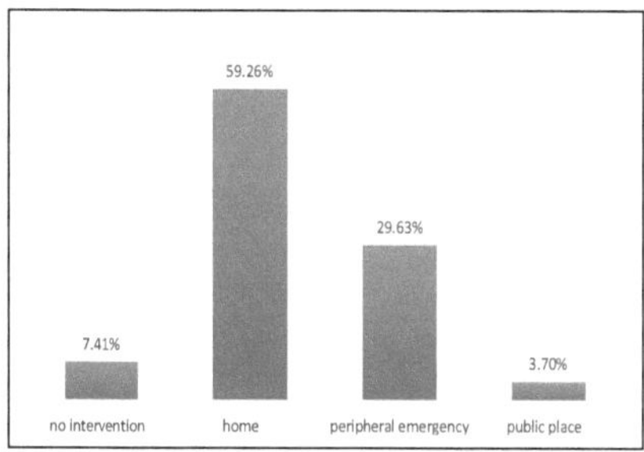

Figure 2: Breakdown of assignments by location

1.2. Patient data

1.2.1. Breakdown by gender

Most of the patients were female (15 cases, 55.6%) and 12 cases were male (44.4%), with a sex ratio of 1.27.

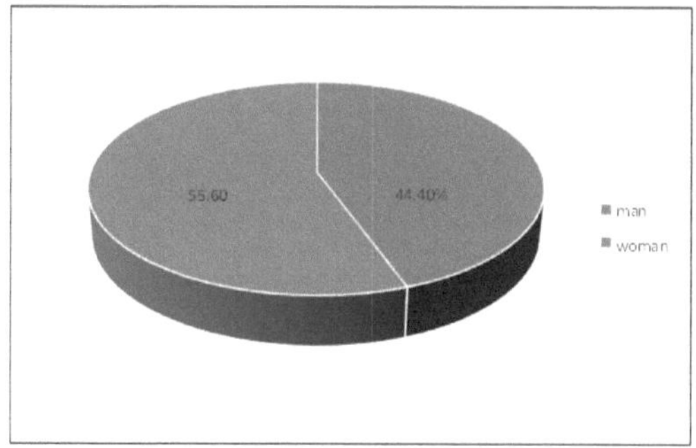

Figure 3: Breakdown of patients by sex

1.2.2. Breakdown by age

The average age of the patients was 75, ranging from 27 to 97. Only one case was aged 27, and the age group most affected was between 60 and 80 (15/27).

Table II: Breakdown by age group :

	Workforce	Percentage (%)
Age [18- 30]	1	3,7
Age [30 - 60]	0	0
Age [60 - 80]	15	55,6
Age ≥ 80 years	11	40,7
Total	27	100

1.2.3. Breakdown by antecedents

Most of the patients, 86.2% (23/27), had a pathological history. Only 4 cases (14.8%) had no previous history.The table below shows the distribution of patients according to history

Table III: Breakdown of patients by medical history :

	Workforce	Percentage (%)
HTA	12/27	44,4
Diabetes	12/27	44,4
Dyslipidemia	10/27	37
Chronic respiratory insufficiency	2/27	7.4
Heart failure	11/27	40.7
Pathology psychiatric	1/27	3.7
AVC	7/27	25.9

1.2.4. Breakdown by lifestyle habits

3 cases (11.1%) were smokers and 18 cases (66.6%) were morbidly obese. Most of the patients were bedridden, i.e. 20 cases (74%), while 6 cases (22.2%) had limited activity. Only one patient was active, aged 27. The average daily water consumption was 1250 ml per 24 hours.

2. Clinical and paraclinical data :

2.1.Clinical data :

The core temperature was high in all patients, with a mean temperature of 40.592 ± 1.579°C and extremes ranging from 38.5 to 43°C. On admission, fatigue was present in 13 cases (48.1%), dizziness in 10 cases (37%), nausea and vomiting in 3 cases (11.1%), muscle cramps in 3 cases (11.1%), headache in 13 cases (48.1%), confusion in 17 cases (63%), syncope in 6 cases (22.2%) and coma in 10 cases (37%). No case presented a convulsive seizure. Signs of dehydration were observed in 44.4% of cases, with a sensation of thirst in 5 cases (18.5%) and dry, erythematous skin in 12 cases (44.4%).

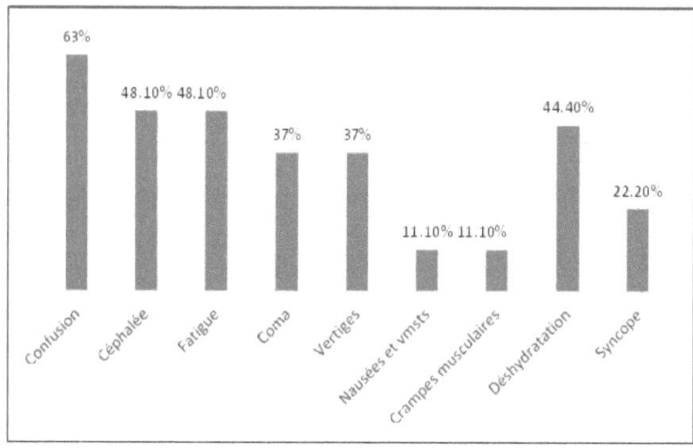

Figure 4: Distribution of patients according to clinical symptoms

On initial examination, neurological disorders were present in most cases (88.9%). 10 cases (37%) were in coma (Glasgow score ≤ 8) with a mean Glasgow score of 8.78 ± 4.2, ranging from 3 to 15. Cardiovascular disorders were present in 81.4% of cases, with arterial hypotension (PAS ≤ 90 mmHg) in 6 cases (22.2%) and tachycardia in 22 cases (81.4%). Arrhythmia was detected by ECG in 13 cases (48.1%).Respiratory distress was observed in more than half the cases (55.5%) with polypnoea (FR ≥ 20 cpm) and increased work of breathing in 8 cases (29.6%) and sa02 hypoxia ≤ 95% in 15 cases (55.5%).

Table IV: Breakdown of clinical constants

Constants	Temperature	NOT	FC	Glasgow	FR	Sp02
Workforce	26/27	26/27	25/27	27/27	25/27	26/27
Mean± Deviation	40,592 ±	121,15 ±	123,56 ±	8,96 ±	23,96 ±	88,62 ±
type	1,5791	37,237	25,138	4,229	4,532	10,127
Maximum	43	190	200	15	34	100
Minimum	38,5	60	80	3	18	65

2.2.Paraclinical data

On a paraclinical level, rhabdomyolysis was noted with increased CPK figures in 4 cases (14.8%), acute renal failure in 9 cases (33.3%), hyperkalaemia $\geq$ 5.5 in 4 cases (14.8%), metabolic acidosis in 4 cases (14.8%) and coagulation disorders in 5 cases (18.5%) with thrombocytopenia in 3 cases (11.1%) and low TP $\leq$ 50% in 5 cases (18.5%).

Table V: Breakdown of biological constants :

Constants	creatinine	urea	TP	platelets	BT	CPK
Workforce	9/27	9/27	5/27	3/27	2/27	4/27
Mean± Deviation type	187,2 ± 34,4	11 ± 4,1	42 ± 4,47	70000 ± 17320	800 ± 3,7	1800 ± 216
Maximum	250	20	50	80000	1000	2000
Minimum	135	6	40	50000	600	1500

3. Therapeutic management

In terms of therapeutic management, 19 cases (70.3%) were placed in a cool area, with 2 cases (7.4%) in the lateral position. 25 cases (92.6%) benefited from rest with physical cooling and 19 cases (70.3%) from pharmacological cooling. Oral hydration was administered in 13 cases (48.1%) and 23 cases (85.1%) received cooled serum filling. 3 cases (11.1%) required the administration of vasoactive drugs to stabilise the haemodynamic state. Oxygen therapy was administered in 13 cases (48.1%), with mechanical ventilation in 6 cases (22.2%).

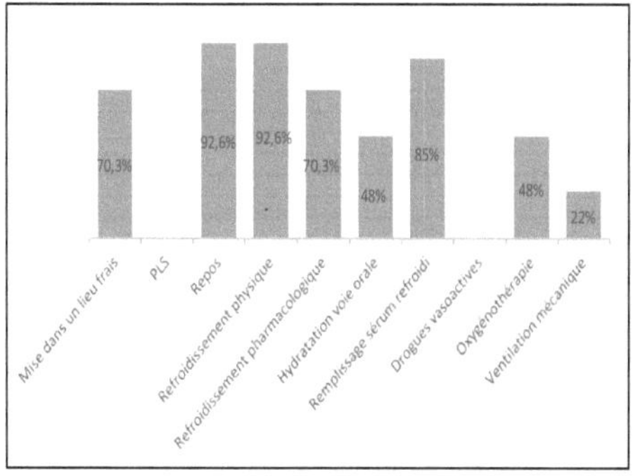

Figure 5: Distribution of patients according to therapeutic management

The average duration of therapeutic management was 99.75+- 48.9 hours, ranging from 45 to 180 hours.

4. Evolution

4.1. Patient destination

Our study concerns 27 victims of heat stroke. 25 cases were treated by the SMUR teams of the centre-east. Regulation decided not to involve the team in two cases, given the unavailability of resources in one case and an incomplete request in the second. 17 cases (62.9%) were transferred to emergency departments (3 cases to the Ibn Jazzar Kairouan emergency department, 5 cases to the Sahloul Sousse emergency department, 5 cases to the Hached Sousse emergency department, 3 cases to the Monastir emergency department and 1 case to the Mahdia emergency department), 1 case (3.7%) was transferred to a private clinic. 6 cases (22.2%) were left at home (4 cases at home and 2 cases in outlying emergency departments).

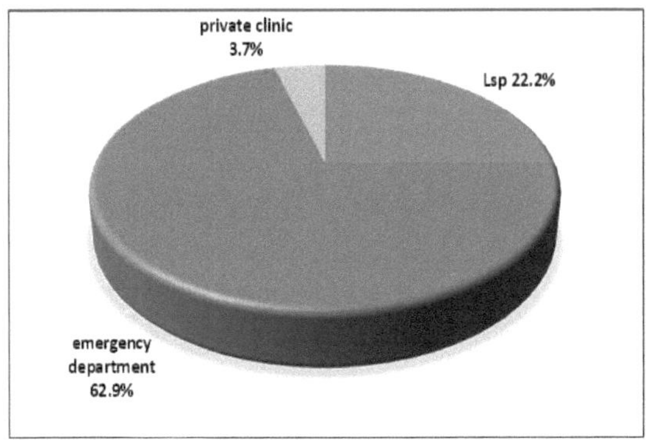

Figure 6: Breakdown of patients by type of care

4.2.Subsequent developments

9/27 cases (33.3%) died and 18/27 cases (66.7%) improved.

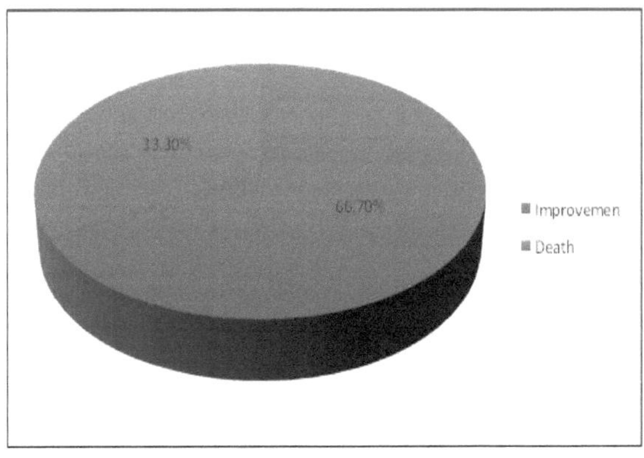

Figure 7: Breakdown of patients by outcome

Improvement was without sequelae in 9 cases and with sequelae in 9 cases. Most of the sequelae were cerebral (8/9). The figure below shows the distribution of patients by sequelae

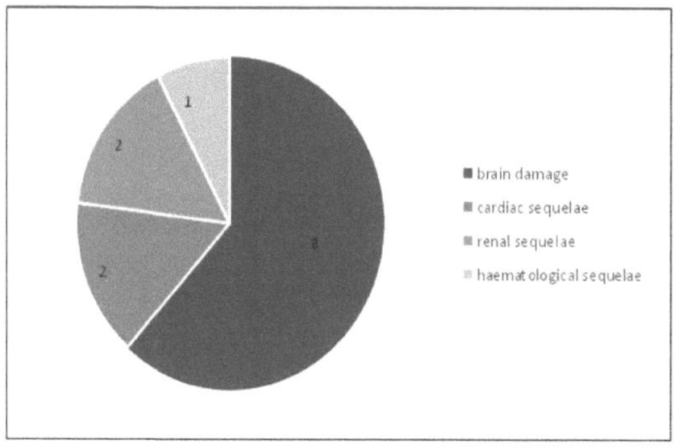

Figure 8: Breakdown of patients by sequelae

The mean time to improvement was 65.37 ± 21.47 hours, with a range of 5 to 100 hours. The average time to death was 11.11 ± 13 hours, ranging from 3 to 45 hours.

II. Analytical study

According to the univariate analysis, the predictive factors of mortality in our study were: central temperature, confusion, coma, visceral damage, haemodynamic distress, acute renal failure, metabolic acidosis, coagulation disorders, rhabdomyolysis, use of VM, drugs, etc. and oral hydration.   No significant difference in cooling.

Table VI: Factors predictive of mortality in our series

	Nombre de cas(%)	Patients décédés n(%)	P
Facteurs épidémiologiques			
Sexe			
Hommes	12 (44,4)	4 (14,8)	0.660
Femmes	15 (55,6)	5(18,5)	
Age			
Inférieur ou égale à 60 ans	1 (3,7)	0(0)	
Entre 60 et 80 ans	15 (55,6)	6(22,2)	0,840
Supérieur ou égale à 80 ans	11(40,7)	3(11,1)	
Antécédents			
Sans ATCDs	4 (14,8)	2 (7,4)	0,444
Avec ATCDs	23 (85,2)	7(25,9)	
Type de SMUR engagée			
Sousse Sahloul	7 (25,9)	2 (7,4)	
Sousse Hached	8 (29,6)	3 (11,1)	
Kairouan	3(11,1)	2(7,4)	
Monastir	5(15,8)	1(3,7)	0,772
Mahdia	1(3,7)	0(0)	
Jam	1(3,7)	0(0)	
Lieu d'intervention			
Pas intervention	2(7,4)	1(3,7)	
A domicile	16(59,3)	4(14,8)	
Urgence périphérique	8(29,6)	4(14,8)	0.522
Lieu publique	1(3,7)	0(0)	
Facteurs d'ordre clinique			
Température centrale			
< 40°C	10 (37)	2(7,4)	0.001
≥ 40°C	17 (63)	7(25,9)	
Céphalée			
Oui	13(48,1)	5(18,5)	0.586
non	14(51,9)	4(14,8)	
Confusion			
Oui	17(63)	2 (7,4)	0.002
non	10(37)	7(25,9)	
Syncope			
Oui	6 (22,2)	1(3,7)	0.326
non	21(77,8)	8(29,6)	
Signes de déshydratation			
Oui	12(44,4)	5(18,5)	0.411
non	15(55,6)	4(14,8)	
Atteinte viscérale			
Oui	20(74,1)	9(33,3)	0.030
non	7(25,9)	0(0)	
Score GCS			
≤8	14 (51,9)	8(29,6)	0.001
>8-15	13(48,1)	1(3,7)	
Détresse respiratoire			
Oui	15(55,5)	2(7,4)	0.242
Non	12(44,4)	7(25,9)	
Détresse hémodynamique			
Oui	6(22,2)	6(22,2)	0.001
Non	21(77,8)	3(11,1)	
Rhabdomyolyse			
Oui	4(14,8)	4(14,8)	0.001
non	23(85,2)	5(18,5)	
Insuffisance rénale aigue			
Oui	9(33,3)	5(18,5)	0.026
Non	18(66,6)	4(14,8)	
Acidose métabolique			
Oui	4(14,8)	4(14,8)	0.001
Non	23(85,2)	5(18,5)	
Troubles de la coagulation			
Oui	5(18,5)	4(14,8)	0.014
non	22(81,5)	5(18,5)	
Facteurs d'ordre thérapeutique			
Recours à la VM			
Oui			0.003
Non	6(22,2)	5(18,5)	
	21(77,8)	4(14,8)	
Oxygénothérapie			
Oui	16(59,3)	7(25,9)	0.166
non	11(40,7)	2(7,4)	
Recours aux catécholamines			
Oui	3(11,1)	3(11,1)	0.009
Non	24(88,9)	6(22,2)	
Refroidissement physique			
Oui	25(92,6)	9(33,3)	0.299
Non	2(7,4)	0(0)	
refroidissement pharmacologique			
oui	19(70,4)	8(29,6)	0.136
non	8(29,6)	1(3,7)	
Hydratation par voie orale			
Oui	13(48,1)	1(3,7)	0.006
non	14(51,9)	8(29,6)	
Remplissage par sérum refroidi			
Oui	23(85,2)	9(33,3)	0.125
non	4(14,8)	0(0)	

DISCUSSION

1. Epidemiological data

Heatstroke is a diagnostic and therapeutic emergency. It is a potentially fatal condition. It is a form of hyperthermia associated with a systemic inflammatory response that leads to a syndrome of multivisceral failure(2).In our study, despite the small sample size, 9 of the 27 cases died. This rate is comparable to other studies in the literature(3,11-14).According to Hifumi et al(3), there were at least 3,332 deaths attributed to heatstroke in the United States between 2006 and 2010.In August 2003, Europe suffered a severe heatwave that lasted nine days and resulted in 14,800 heat-related deaths in France, including 2,800 cases attributed to heat stroke, the most serious form of heat illness (1).Several studies have described the characteristics of the victims of this heatwave.The study by Argaud et al (14) looked at 83 cases of heat stroke admitted to a university hospital in Lyon and showed that the mortality rates at 28 days and 2 years were 58% and 71% respectively.The study by Pease et al(11) is a cohort study of 22 heatstroke victims hospitalised in intensive care units and showed that the mortality rate was 63.6%.According to studies(1,3,4,14), the number of deaths due to heatstroke is expected to increase in subsequent years as a result of climate change and global warming. According to Argoud et al(14), by the 2050s, heatstroke-related deaths are expected to increase by almost 2.5 times the current annual baseline of around 2,000 deaths.Despite this high mortality rate, heat stroke has not been studied in depth for several possible reasons. Firstly, although sepsis, acute respiratory distress syndrome (ARDS) and acute renal failure (ARF) include simple and commonly used definitions, no universally accepted definition of heatstroke exists in the clinical setting(3). Secondly, because large numbers of heatstroke victims are rare in the United States or European countries (e.g. 1995 and 1999 in Chicago, 2003 in Paris) (13-16), clinical research has not been carried out on an ongoing basis in these regions(3).In our study, most of the patients were female, 15 cases (55.6%), and 12 cases were male (44.4%), with a sex ratio of 1.27. The mean age of the patients was 75 years, ranging from 27 to 97 years. Only one case, aged 27, was the most affected age group.was between 60 and 80 years of age (15/27). Most of the patients (86.2%, 23/27) had a pathological history. 44.4% (12/27) had hypertension. 7.4% (2/27) had a chronic respiratory disease. 3.7% (1/27) had a psychiatric condition. 40.7% (11/27) had chronic heart failure. Most of the patients were bedridden, i.e. 20 cases (74%), 6 cases (22.2%) had limited activity. Only one subject was active, aged 27. This is comparable to the results in the literature(11,14).In the study by Pease et al(11), the sex ratio of patients was 1, with a median age of 68.5 years (61.3-76.8). 91% of patients had a pathological history. 36% (8/22) had psychiatric disorders, 45% (10/22) were hypertensive, 23% (5/22) had chronic respiratory disease (asthma, COPD) and 1 patient had a history of pheochromocytoma.In the study by Argaud et al(14), seventy patients (84%) were elderly (>70 years), 29 cases (41%) lived in institutions and 48 (69%) had limited physical activity. Twenty-seven patients (33%) were aged 85 or over. Of all the patients, 80 (96%) had a pathological history and 63 (76%) were being treated with an antihypertensive drug (mainly diuretics) and/or a neurotropic drug (mainly tranquillisers).

2. Clinical and paraclinical data

Excessive exposure to heat leads to thermoregulatory failure. Appearing at rest during heat waves, heatstroke manifests itself as neurological and cardiovascular distress and, if left untreated, can progress to multivisceral failure syndrome(3).

In fact, the definition of heatstroke most commonly used around the world is that of Bouchama(2). Bouchama defined heatstroke as a core body temperature in excess of 40°C, accompanied by signs of dehydration and central nervous system abnormalities such as delirium, convulsions or coma(2,3).The second definition is based on the physiopathology of heatstroke, which results from a failure of thermoregulation coupled with an exaggeration of the thermal immuno-inflammatory response and a poor response from heat shock proteins(1,2). The complex interaction between the physiological changes caused by hyperthermia, the cytotoxic effect of heat, and the host's immuno-inflammatory and haemostatic response results in the onset of the multivisceral failure syndrome, principally encephalopathy(1,2).Pease et al(11) referred to the following criteria in their study according to Bouchama's definition: altered neurological state (coma, delirium, disorientation or convulsions); a core temperature > 40.6°C; a a reliable history of compatible environmental exposure; and the presence of warm, dry or reddened skin. In another study, Misset et al(17) defined heat stroke as "the presence of hyperthermia > 40.5°C" but the term "core body temperature" was not included in their definition. As a result, the specific body temperature and the use of the term "core body temperature" vary between studies(2,11,17).In our study, the temperature was high in all patients, with a mean core temperature of 40.592 ± 1.579 and extremities ranging from 38.5 to 43°C, which is comparable to other studies. In the study by Argaud et al(14), thirty-nine patients (47%) had a temperature greater than or equal to 41°C. In the study by Pease et al(11), the median core temperature on admission was 41.1°C. In our study, neurological disorders were present in most cases (88.9%). 14 cases (51.9%) were in coma, with an average Glasgow score of 9 ± 4.2 and extremities ranging from 3 to 15. Cardiovascular disorders were present in 81.4% of cases, with arterial hypotension (PAS ≤ 90 mmHg) in 6 cases (22.2%) and tachycardia in 22 cases (81.4%). Arrhythmia was detected by ECG in 13 cases (48.1%). Signs of dehydration were observed in 44.4% of cases, with a sensation of thirst in 5 cases (18.5%) and dry, erythematous skin in 12.cases (44.4%). Respiratory distress was observed in more than half the cases (55.5%). Biologically, rhabdomyolysis was noted in 4 cases (14.8%), acute renal failure in 9 cases (33.3%) with a mean creatinine level of 187.2 ± 34.4 (135-250), hyperkalaemia ≥ 5,5 in 4 cases (14.8%), metabolic acidosis in 4 cases (14.8%) and coagulation disorders in 5 cases (18.5%) with thrombocytopenia in 3 cases (11.1%) with a mean platelet count of70000 ± 17320(50000-80000). The PT was low ≤ 50% in 5 cases (18.5%) with a mean PT of 42 ± 4.47 (40-50). These clinical and paraclinical data were comparable with the results of other studies(11,13,14). In the study by Dematte et al(13) carried out in Chicago, 58 patients were admitted to hospital during the 1995 heat wave. The patients presented with multi-organ dysfunction with neurological impairment in 100% of cases, moderate to severe renal failure in 53% of cases, disseminated intravascular coagulation in 45% of cases and acute respiratory distress syndrome in 10%. In the study by Pease et al(11), all patients presented with neurological, respiratory and cardiac visceral involvement. On admission, the mean Glasgow score was 10 with a range of 3 to 15. All patients had renal, hepatic and haematological involvement. The rate of Creatinine, mean was 119 (102-173), Bilirubin mean 12 (10-20), mean platelet count 133 (72-196) and CPK 771 (143-3,215).In the study by Argaud et al(14) , 47 cases (57%) presented a coma, 36 cases (43 %) were in shock and 19 cases (23%) had anuria. In addition to ongoing neurological dysfunction, 53 patients (66%) had at least one additional organ failure. Mean creatinine and urea nitrogen values were slightly elevated: 1.76 ± 0.93 mg/dL and 39.50 ± 23.53 mg/dL, respectively. When blood gases and pH were analysed (45 patients), respiratory alkalosis was found in 23 patients (51%) and metabolic acidosis in 12 patients (27%). Mean arterial pressure ± SD in oxygen was 75 ± 39 mm Hg. Creatinine kinase levels were above twice the normal limit in 45 patients (54%). Electrocardiography revealed ischaemic abnormalities in 30 patients (36%); these were confirmed by an increase in troponin I levels in 20 patients (29%). Twenty-five patients (40%) had hepatic cytolysis without cholestasis. Thrombocytopenia (thrombocyte count, $95 ± 37 × 10\ 3\ /\mu L$) and a low prothrombin index (53% ± 16%) were detected in 23 (28%) and 30 (36%) patients, respectively.

3. Therapeutic management

According to the literature(4,6,11,14), cooling is the gold standard in the management of patients suffering from heatstroke. Ice water immersion has been shown to be highly effective in the treatment of exertional heatstroke, with a zero mortality rate in a large series of cases of younger, physically fit patients. In elderly patients suffering from non-exertional heatstroke, studies have more often favoured evaporative and convective cooling. Evaporative and convective cooling can be augmented by crushed ice or ice packs applied diffusely over the body. Refrigerated intravenous fluids can also supplement primary cooling(4).

Based on current evidence, ice packs are applied strategically to the neck, armpits and groin; cooling blankets; and intravascular or external cooling devices are not recommended as primary cooling methods in heat stroke(4).

According to studies(4,6), aggressive cooling should be administered as quickly as possible to patients suffering from heatstroke in order to avoid the onset of neurological sequelae.In our study, 19 cases (70.3%) were placed in a cool area, with 2 cases (7.4%) in the lateral position. 25 cases (92.6%) benefited from rest with physical cooling and 19 cases (70.3%) from pharmacological cooling. Oral hydration was administered in 13 cases. (48.1%) and 23 cases (85.1%) benefited from cooled serum filling. 3 cases (11.1%) required the administration of vasoactive drugs to stabilise the haemodynamic state. Oxygen therapy was provided in 13 cases (48.1%), with mechanical ventilation in 6 cases (22.2%). This is comparable to the results of other studies(4,11,14). In the study by Argaud et al(14), in addition to symptomatic care related to their organ dysfunction (including, if necessary, mechanical ventilation, vasoactive and/or inotropic agents and volume expansion), all patients received a liquid infusion

(2.5 ± 1.0 L during the first 24 hours), and 79 (95%) received antipyretic agents (acetaminophen). External cooling was performed on only 41 patients (49%).

4. Evolution

In our study, 9/27 cases (33.3%) died and 18/27 cases (66.7%) improved. Improvement was without sequelae in 9 cases and with sequelae in 9 cases. Most of the sequelae were cerebral (8/9). 2 cases had cardiac sequelae, 2 had renal sequelae and one had haematological sequelae. This was comparable to the results of other studies(11,13,14).In the study by Dematte et al(13), in-hospital mortality was 21%. Most of the survivors recovered an almost normal renal, haematological and respiratory status, but the disability persisted, leading to an impairment moderate to severe functional impairment in 33% of patients at discharge. At 1 year, none of the patients had improved their functional status and 28% of the additional patients had died.In the study by Pease et al(11), mortality was 63.6% (14/22). 7 patients died within the first 7 days following multivisceral failure and 7 cases died with neurological sequelae (coma = 6, tetraplegia = 1). The median total length of hospital stay was 17 days (2-25.5), and after discharge from the intensive care unit no patient died during a one-year follow-up.

5. Factors predictive of mortality

In our study, the factors predictive of mortality were: core temperature, confusion, coma, visceral damage, haemodynamic distress, acute renal failure, metabolic acidosis, coagulation disorders, rhabdomyolysis, use of MV, vasoactive drugs and oral hydration. There was no significant difference in cooling. These results were comparable to those reported in the literature(14,17,18).In the study by Argaud et al(14), demographic characteristics (i.e. age and sex) were not significantly different between survivors and deaths on day 28. However, the factors predictive of death were: long-term use of antihypertensive drugs (P = 0.004) or phenothiazine-based drugs (P = 0.02), coma (P < 0.001), anuria (P < 0.001), and the presence of anaemia (P < 0.001). (P < 0.001), metabolic acidosis (P = 0.001). No differences in heatstroke-related treatment, such as cooling, antipyretic agents or fluid infusion, were observed between survivors and deaths. The multivariate Cox proportional hazards model revealed an independent contribution to mortality if patients were on long-term antihypertensive medication or presented on admission with cardiovascular failure, anuria or coma.The study by Hausfater et al(18) included all patients with a core temperature > 38.5°C admitted to one of the emergency departments during the heatwave of August 2003 in Paris. According to this study, the predictive factors for mortality from heat stroke without exertion were: previous treatment with diuretics, a stay in an institution, age > 80 years, history of chronic heart failure or neoplasia, core temperature > 40°C, systolic blood pressure < 100 mmHg, GSC scale < 12, and transport to hospital by ambulance.Misset et al(17) conducted a multivariate analysis looking at the occurrence of heatstroke at home or in a healthcare institution (vs. in a public place). This study showed that the presence of a high initial body temperature, a prolonged prothrombin time, the use of vasoactive drugs during the first day in an intensive care unit, etc. were all associated with the occurrence of heatstroke. (ICU) and managing patients in an ICU without air conditioning were associated with a significant risk of in-hospital death. The Hifumi et al(3) study of 705 heatstroke patients found that in-hospital mortality was 7.1% (50 patients). Multiple regression analysis revealed that in-hospital mortality was significantly associated with PAS (odds ratio (OR): 0.99; 95% CI [0.98 to 0.99] with p = 0.026) the GCS score (OR, 0.77; 95% CI [0.69 0.86] with p < 0.01), serum creatinine levels (OR: 1.28; 95% CI: [1.02-1.61]; p = 0.032) and the presence of DIC on admission (OR: 2.16; 95% CI: [1.09-4.27]; p = 0.028).

STRENGTHS AND LIMITATIONS OF THE STUDY

1. Highlights

Our work is interesting because it is one of the few studies and the first to be carried out in Tunisia on a relevant and common subject, heatstroke. In fact, our study offers a significant contribution to the understanding of heat stroke in Tunisia, laying the foundations for continued improvements in the prevention, diagnosis and management of this critical condition. These advances are essential to ensure an effective medical response to this growing climatic emergency.

2. Limitations of the study :

- Despite the lessons learned from this study, certain limitations must be taken into account, such as the size of the sample and the duration of the study.

- Given the small sample size of our study (27 cases), multivariate analysis was not possible.

- Future research could extend these investigations to a national scale and over a longer period to consolidate our conclusions.

CONCLUSION

Heat stroke is a major public health problem. It is a major cause of mortality and morbidity. It is a form of hyperthermia associated with a systemic inflammatory response that leads to a syndrome of multivisceral failure(2).Given the seriousness of this climatic emergency, the involvement of medical teams in the pre-hospital phase of the care of these patients is fundamental to improving the effectiveness of care and limiting the after-effects of heatstroke. Our study was carried out in the territory of the SAMU 03 of Tunisia during the heat wave of the year 2023. More than half of the patients in our study were female, i.e. 15/27 cases (55.6%) with a sex ratio of 1.27. The average age of the patients was 75 years, ranging from 27 to 97 years. Clinically, the core temperature was high in all patients, with a mean temperature of 40.592 ± 1.579 [38.5-43°C], and neurological disorders were present in most cases (88.9%). Cardiovascular disorders were present in 81.4% of cases. Signs of dehydration were observed in 44.4% of cases, and respiratory distress was observed in more than half (55.5%). 25 cases (92.6%) benefited from physical cooling and 19 cases (70.3%) from pharmacological cooling. Oral hydration was administered in 13 cases.(48.1%) and 23 cases (85.1%) benefited from cooled serum filling. 3 cases (11.1%) required the administration of vasoactive drugs. Oxygen therapy was provided in 13 cases (48.1%), with mechanical ventilation in 6 cases (22.2%). In terms of evolution, 9/27 cases (33.3%) died and 18/27 cases (66.7%) improved. Improvement was without sequelae in 9 cases and with sequelae in 9 cases. Most of the sequelae were cerebral (8/9). 2 cases had cardiac sequelae, 2 had renal sequelae and one had haematological sequelae. Factors predictive of mortality according to univariate analysis were: central temperature, confusion, coma, visceral damage, haemodynamic distress, acute renal failure, metabolic acidosis, coagulation disorders, rhabdomyolysis, use of VM, vasoactive drugs and oral hydration. No significant difference in cooling. The literature

(3,11,13,14,17) and our study have shown that the mortality rate following heatstroke is significant, and even if cooling procedures and intensive care management are rapidly initiated, classic heatstroke can result in rapid worsening of organ dysfunction leading to death. Hence the need for more in-depth studies in this context in order to improve the means of therapeutic management.

REFERENCES

1. Rahmoune C, Bouchama A. Heat stroke. Réanimation. May 2004;13(3):190-6.

2. Bouchama A, Knochel JP. Heat stroke. N Engl J Med. 20 June 2002;346(25):1978-88.

3. Hifumi T, Kondo Y, Shimizu K, Miyake Y. Heat stroke. J Intensive Care.22 May 2018;6(1):30.

4. Gaudio FG, Grissom CK. Cooling Methods in Heat Stroke. J Emerg Med. Apr 2016;50(4):607-16.

5. Gazzah DM. The Glasgow score.

6. Nakamura S. [Sequelae secondary to heat-related illness]. Nihon Rinsho Jpn J Clin Med. June 2012;70(6):969-74.

7. Yumoto T, Naito H, Yorifuji T, Aokage T, Fujisaki N, Nakao A. Association of Japan Coma Scale score on hospital arrival with in-hospital mortality among trauma patients. BMC Emerg Med. Nov 6, 2019;19(1):65.

8. Singh RK, Baronia AK, Sahoo JN, Sharma S, Naval R, Pandey CM, et al.Prospective comparison of new Japanese Association for Acute Medicine (JAAM) DIC and International Society of Thrombosis and Hemostasis (ISTH) DIC score in critically ill septic patients. Thromb Res. 1 Apr 2012;129(4):e119-25.

9. Gando S, Saitoh D, Ogura H, Mayumi T, Koseki K, Ikeda T, et al. Disseminated intravascular coagulation (DIC) diagnosed based on the Japanese Association for Acute Medicine criteria is a dependent continuum to overt DIC in patients with sepsis. Thromb Res. 1 March 2009;123(5):715-8.

10. Hifumi T, Kondo Y, Shimazaki J, Oda Y, Shiraishi S, Wakasugi M, et al.

Prognostic significance of disseminated intravascular coagulation in patients with heat stroke in a nationwide registry. J Crit Care. Apr 2018;44:306-11.

11. Pease S, Bouadma L, Kermarrec N, Schortgen F, Régnier B, Wolff M. Early organ dysfunction course, cooling time and outcome in classic heatstroke. Intensive Care Med. August 2009;35(8):1454-8.

12. Naughton MP, Henderson A, Mirabelli MC, Kaiser R, Wilhelm JL, Kieszak SM, et al. Heat-related mortality during a 1999 heat wave in Chicago. Am J Prev Med. May 2002;22(4):221-7.

13. Dematte JE, O'Mara K, Buescher J, Whitney CG, Forsythe S, McNamee T, et al. Near-Fatal Heat Stroke during the 1995 Heat Wave in Chicago. Ann Intern Med. August 1998;129(3):173-81.

14. Argaud L, Ferry T, Le QH, Marfisi A, Ciorba D, Achache P, et al. Short- and long-term outcomes of heatstroke following the 2003 heat wave in Lyon, France. Arch Intern Med. 12 Nov 2007;167(20):2177-83.

15. Naughton MP, Henderson A, Mirabelli MC, Kaiser R, Wilhelm JL, Kieszak SM, et al. Heat-related mortality during a 1999 heat wave in Chicago1. Am J Prev Med. 1 May 2002;22(4):221-7.

16. Semenza JC, Rubin CH, Falter KH, Selanikio JD, Flanders WD, Howe HL, et al. Heat-related deaths during the July 1995 heat wave in Chicago. N Engl J Med. July 11, 1996;335(2):84-90.

17. Misset B, De Jonghe B, Bastuji-Garin S, Gattolliat O, Boughrara E, Annane D, et al. Mortality of patients with heatstroke admitted to intensive care units during the 2003 heat wave in France: A national multiple-center risk-factor study*. Crit Care Med. Apr 2006;34(4):1087.

18. Hausfater P, Megarbane B, Dautheville S, Patzak A, Andronikof M, Santin A, et al. Prognostic factors in non-exertional heatstroke. Intensive Care Med. Feb 2010;36(2):272-80.

APPENDICES

Appendix 1: Data collection form: Heat stroke

I. Epidemiological data :

- Date: ... /... /...... ; Time: ... : ... ;

- Ambient temperature at time of call: ... °C

- Full name: ....

- Mission data :

1. Appeal Governorate (Sousse Monastir Kairouan Mahdia)

2. Reason for call: disturbed consciousness □ dyspnoea + disturbed consciousness □ haemodynamic instability + disturbed consciousness □

3. Regulation decision: to engage the team □ or not □

4. SMUR engaged: Kairouan □ Sousse □ Monastir □ Mahdia □ Jam □

5. Type of mission: primary □ primary-secondary □ secondary □

6. The place of intervention: home □ public place □ peripheral emergency □

- Patient data :

1. gender: Male □Female □

2. Age: ... years

3. History Diabetes □ High blood pressure □ Dyslipidemia □ Respiratory disease □ Cardiac disease □ History of stroke □ Psychiatric disease □

4. Daily physical activity: active bedridden limited physical activity

5. Lifestyle habits: smoking, alcohol, obesity,

6. Average water consumption per 24 hours.

II. Clinical Data :

1- Symptomatology: Fever □ Headache □ Confusion □Nausea/Vomiting □Dry, hot skin □ Feeling thirsty □ Signs of dehydration □ Muscle cramp □ Fatigue □ Vertigo □Syncope □Coma □

3- Parameters: GCS:....BP: ....mmHg: .... bpm FR: .... c/mn SaO2: .... %: C°

Breathing work

Ventilation:

6- ECG :

III. Biology :

Hb: ...... Ht: ...... GB: ...... Plq: ...... TP: ......INR: .....   TCK: .....

Na+: ...... K+: ...... Cl-: ...... Urea: ...... Creat: ......

ASAT : ...... ALAT : ...... BT : ...... BD : ...... CPK : ...... LDH : ......

Ca: ..... P : ....

IV. Therapeutic management :

1- Duration of treatment: .... hours

2- Put in a cooler place: No □ Yes □

3- Rest: No □ Yes □

4- Physical cooling: No □ Yes □

5- Pharmacological cooling: No □ Yes □

6- Oral hydration: No □ Yes □

7- Filling cooled serum

8- PLS: No □ Yes □

9- Use of anti-inflammatory drugs: No □ Yes □

10- Oxygen therapy: No □ Yes □

11- Respiratory assistance: No □ Yes □

12- Vasoactive drugs: No □ Yes □

V.Evolution :

1- Place of orientation :

2- Improvement without sequelae: No □ Yes □, if Yes improvement after: ....
hours

3- Initial visceral damage: No □ Yes □

If yes: Cerebral □ Cardiac □ Hepatic □ Renal □ Haematological □ 4- Remaining
sequelae : No □ Yes □

If yes: Cerebral □ Cardiac □ Hepatic □ Renal □ Haematological □ 5- Death: No
□ Yes □

Duration of care before improvement: ... hours Duration of care before death: ....
hours

Appendix 2: Glasgow score (5)

Valeur	GCS adulte
Ouverture des yeux	
4	Ouverture spontanée
3	Ouverture à la commande verbale
2	Ouverture à la stimulation douloureuse
1	Pas d'ouverture des yeux
Réponse verbale	
5	Réponse orientée
4	Conversation confuse
3	Mots inappropriés
2	Sons incompréhensibles
1	Pas de réponse verbale
Réponse motrice	
6	Obéit aux commandes
5	Localise la douleur
4	Retrait à la douleur
3	Flexion anormale à la douleur
2	Extension à la douleur
1	Pas de réponse motrice

Appendix 3: Diagnostic criteria for heat stroke according to JAAM (3)

Classification recommended by the Japanese Association of Acute Medicine "Committee related to heatstroke"

Japanese Association of Acute Medicine Heat Related Illness Classification 2015

	Symptoms	Severity	Treatment	Classification from clinical presentations
Stage I (First aid and observation)	Dizziness, faintness, slight yawning Heavy sweating Muscle pain, stiff muscles (muscle cramps) Impaired consciousness is not observed (JCS = 0)		May be handled on site under normal conditions → Resting in a cool place, cooling the body surface, and orally supplying water and Na	Heat cramp Heat syncope
Stage II (Should be taken to a medical institution)	Headache, vomiting, fatigue, sinking feeling, and declined concentration and judgement (JCS ≤ 1)		Examination at a medical institution is necessary → Body temperature management, resting, and sufficiently supplying water and Na⁺ (by drip infusion if oral intake is difficult)	Heat exhaustion
Stage III (Inpatient hospital care)	Includes at least one of the following: (C) central nervous system manifestation (impaired consciousness JCS ≥ 2, cerebellar symptoms, convulsive seizures) (H/K) hepatic/renal dysfunction (follow-up following admission to hospital, hepatic or renal impairment requiring inpatient hospital care) - - - - - - - - - - (D) Coagulation disorder (diagnosed as DIC according to acute phase DIC diagnostic criteria (Japanese Association of Acute Medicine) → Most severe of the three types		Inpatient hospital care (depending on the case, intensive care) is necessary → Body temperature management (internal body cooling, intravascular cooling, etc. are carried out along with body surface cooling) Respiratory and circulatory care DIC treatment	Heat stroke

Appendix 4: Japanese coma scale (7)

Figure 1: Japan Coma Scale Scoring

0: Clear

1: Almost fully conscious

2: Unable to recognize time, place and person

3: Unable to recall name or DOB

10: Rousable by being spoken to but reverts to previous state if stimulus stops

20: Rousable with loud voice but reverts to previous state if stimulus stops

30: Rousable only by repeated mechanical stimuli

100: Unrousable using any forceful stimuli but responds to avoid the stimuli

200: Unrousable using any forceful stimuli but responds with slight movements, including decerebrate or decorticate postures

300: Unrousable using any forceful stimuli and does not respond at all

Appendix 5: Disseminated intravascular coagulation (DIC) score according to JAAM (3,8,9)

	Score
Systemic inflammatory response syndrome criteria	
≥ 3	1
0–2	0
Platelet count (150×109 /L)	
<80 or >50% decrease within 24 hours	3
≥ 80 and <120 or >30% decrease within 24 hours	1
≥ 120	0
Prothrombin time (value of patient/normal value)	
≥ 1.2	1
<1.2	0
Fibrin/fibrinogen degradation products (mg/L)	
≥ 25	3
≥ 10 and <25	1
<10	0
Diagnosis	
Four points or more	DIC

Appendix 6: The difference in definitions/classifications of heat stroke between the Bouchama definition and the JAAM and JAAM-HS-WG criteria (3)

		Bouchama's definition	JAAM criteria	JAAM-HS-WG criteria
Environment		Exposure to ambient heat (classic heat stroke)	Exposure to high environmental temperatures	
Body temperature		Core body temperature > 40 °C	-	-
Organ dysfunction	Central nervous system	Delirium, convulsions or coma	Disturbed consciousness JCS ≥ 2, cerebellar symptoms, convulsions	GCS score ≤ 14
	Coagulation	-	Diagnosed as DIC by JAAM	JAAM DIC score ≥ 4
	Liver	-	Follow-up after hospitalisation, liver or kidney failure requiring hospitalisation	Creatinine or total bilirubin levels ≥ 1.2 mg/dL
	Renal	-		
	Cardiovascular	-	-	-
	Respiratory	-	-	-

SUMMARY

Introduction: *Heat stroke is a life-threatening medical emergency. It is defined by the combination of a rapid rise in core temperature above 40 °C and neurological (delirium, convulsions or coma) and cardiovascular disorders. This can lead to multivisceral failure syndrome and death.*

Objectives: *To describe the clinical, therapeutic and prognostic features of heatstroke and determine the factors predictive of mortality.*

Patients and methods*: Our work is a descriptive cross-sectional study of 27 heatstroke victims treated pre-hospital by the SAMU 03 service of the centre-east, over a period of 3 months (June-August 2023).*

Results: *In our study, most of the patients were female, i.e. 15/27 cases (55.6%) with a sex ratio of 1.27. The average age of the patients was 75 years, ranging from 27 to 97 years. Most of the patients (86.2%, 23/27) had a pathological history. Clinically, the core temperature was high in all patients, with a mean temperature of 40.592 ± 1.579 [38.5-43°C]. Neurological disorders were present in most cases (88.9%). 14 cases (51.9%) were in coma, with a mean Glasgow score of 9 ± 4.2. Cardiovascular disorders were present in 81.4% of cases, with arterial hypotension (PAS ≤ 90 mmHg) in 6 cases (22.2%). Signs of dehydration were observed in 44.4% of cases, and respiratory distress was observed in more than half the cases (55.5%). Biologically, rhabdomyolysis was noted in 4 cases (14.8%), acute renal failure in 9 cases (33.3%), metabolic acidosis in 4 cases (14.8%) and coagulation disorders in 5 cases (18.5%). With regard to therapeutic management, 25 cases (92.6%) benefited from physical cooling and 19 cases (70.3%) from pharmacological cooling. Oral hydration was administered in 13 cases (48.1%) and 23 cases (85.1%) received cooled serum filling. 3 cases (11.1%) required the administration of vasoactive drugs. Oxygen therapy was provided in 13 cases (48.1%), with mechanical ventilation* *in 6 cases (22.2%). In terms of evolution, 9/27 cases (33.3%) died and 18/27 cases (66.7%) improved. Improvement was without sequelae in 9 cases and with sequelae in 9 cases. Most of the sequelae were cerebral (8/9). 2 cases had cardiac sequelae, 2 had renal sequelae and one had haematological sequelae. According to the univariate analysis, the factors predictive of mortality were: central temperature, confusion, coma, visceral damage, haemodynamic distress, acute renal failure, metabolic acidosis, coagulation disorders, rhabdomyolysis, use of VM, vasoactive drugs and oral hydration. No significant difference in cooling.*

Conclusion: *Heat stroke is a major public health problem. It is a major cause of mortality and morbidity. The involvement of medical teams in the pre-hospital phase of the management of these patients is fundamental to improving the effectiveness of care and limiting the after-effects of heatstroke.*

Key words: *heat stroke, pre-hospital care, treatment, mortality*

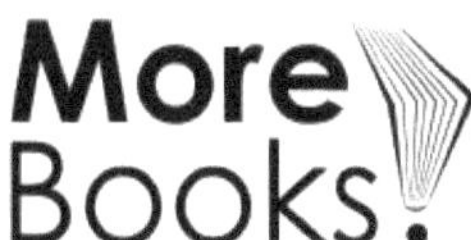

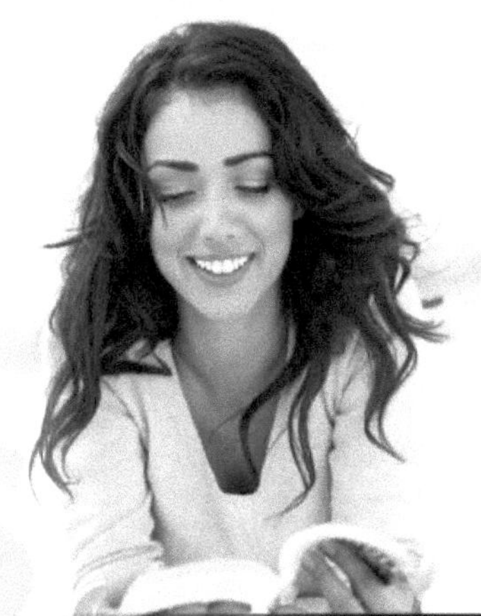

I want morebooks!

Buy your books fast and straightforward online - at one of world's fastest growing online book stores! Environmentally sound due to Print-on-Demand technologies.

Buy your books online at
www.morebooks.shop

Kaufen Sie Ihre Bücher schnell und unkompliziert online – auf einer der am schnellsten wachsenden Buchhandelsplattformen weltweit! Dank Print-On-Demand umwelt- und ressourcenschonend produziert.

Bücher schneller online kaufen
www.morebooks.shop

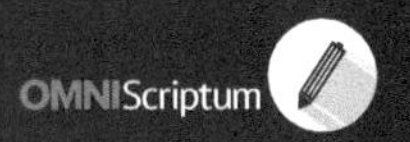

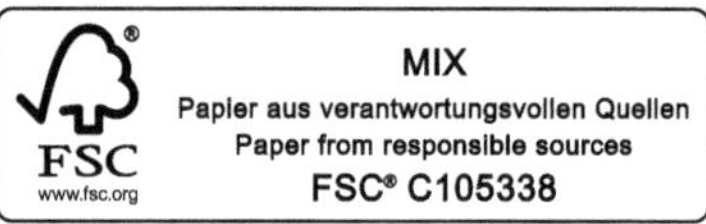

Printed by Books on Demand GmbH, Norderstedt / Germany